Mustapha Benmahdjoub

Behçet's disease

Mustapha Benmahdjoub

Behçet's disease

Systemic manifestations

ScienciaScripts

Imprint

Cover image: www.ingimage.com

This book is a translation from the original published under ISBN 978-620-6-71550-4.

Publisher:
Sciencia Scripts
is a trademark of
Dodo Books Indian Ocean Ltd. and OmniScriptum S.R.L publishing group

120 High Road, East Finchley, London, N2 9ED, United Kingdom
Str. Armeneasca 28/1, office 1, Chisinau MD-2012, Republic of Moldova, Europe
Printed at: see last page
ISBN: 978-620-7-75652-0

BEHÇET'S DISEASE.

SYSTEMIC MANIFESTATIONS

AUTHORS: M. BENMAHDJOUB.

TABLE OF CONTENTS

SUMMARY

Behçet's disease (BD) is a multi-systemic, autoimmune vasculitis characterized by a broad clinical spectrum including recurrent bipolar (oral and genital) ulcerations associated with ocular, neurological, cutaneous, vascular, digestive and other manifestations. joints. This condition affects both men and women between the ages of 20 and 40. It is relatively common in the Mediterranean basin and the Far East. This condition should be suspected when the process is severe and/or recurrent, and that the patient is from a highly endemic area. There is no biological marker that can be used to establish a definitive diagnosis. Diagnosis is based on clinical criteria that are constantly being revised.

The neurological manifestations of MB are dominated by parenchymal involvement, with variable clinical presentation.Magnetic resonance imaging (MRI) of the brain is the gold standard for this condition. Management of MB is guided by the severity of the disease and the type of organ affected. In general, colchicine, non-steroidal anti-inflammatory drugs (NSAIDs) and corticosteroids are often sufficient to control the mucocutaneous and articular manifestations of MB. Involvement of other organs, particularly neurological, ocular and gastrointestinal, which may be life-threatening or functionally impaired, requires a more aggressive strategy from the outset, with immunosuppressive drugs. Therapeutic advances with the development of new molecules, immunomodulators (anti-TNFα and interferon), therapies targeting lymphocytes (Anti-CD20, Anti-CD52, Anti-CD25 and haematopoietic stem cell autografts) have improved the prognosis of this disease.

Key words: *Behçet's disease, Systemic manifestations, Diagnostic criteria, Cerebral imaging, Treatment.*

I) INTRODUCTION

Behçet's disease (BD) is a multi-systemic autoimmune vasculitis characterised by a broad clinical spectrum including recurrent bipolar ulcerations (oral and genital), associated with ocular, neurological, cutaneous, vascular, digestive and articular manifestations [1,2] . On the one hand, it is a dreaded disease because of its neurological and ocular complications, which can lead to functional and life-threatening sequelae.

arterial complications, which are rare but also cause increased mortality[3] . In the absence of biological markers, MB is diagnosed clinically on the basis of criteria that are regularly re-evaluated [4,5,6] . Treatment is essentially symptomatic, which has improved long-term functional and vital prognosis[7] .

II) HISTORY

The first description of MB seems to date back to Hippocrates in the 5th century BC, 2,500 years ago. In the Third Book of Epidemic Diseases, he describes this clinical entity as an endemic disease occurring in Asia Minor, characterised by "aphthous ulcerations", "defluxions of the genitals" and "chronic aqueous ophthalmic involvement causing many people to lose their sight" [(8,9, 10)]. Thereafter, no description in medical literature was noted until the 20ème century. In 1931, Amantiadès (a Greek ophthalmologist) published a case with: oral-genital ulcerations, iritis with hypopion and hydarthrosis. 6 years later, Huluci Behçet (1937), a Turkish dermatologist, identified the classic triad associating uveitis with hypopion, oral and genital aphtosis[(11)] . Since then, his name has become the eponym for this condition.

III) EPIDEMIOLOGY

MB is thought to have developed in countries around the Mediterranean, across Asia and as far as Japan, following the silk route used by nomadic or Turkic tribes (Fig 1). Descriptive epidemiological data largely support the hypothesis of a geographical disparity in the frequency of occurrence of MB. The name "Silk Road disease" is linked to the high incidence of the condition in these areas, and has given rise to the hypothesis that the aetiological agent of MB was carried by this ancient merchant route. This geographical distribution is highlighted by the association of MB with carriage of the same HLA allele in the different ethnic groups studied(12) .

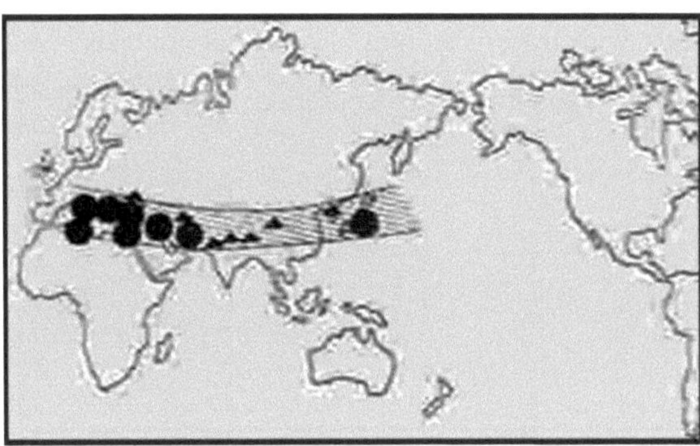

Figure 1: The Silk Road used by nomadic tribes.

1°) Prevalence :

The epidemiological aspects of MB have their own particularities, notably its geographical distribution (Fig 2). MB is very common in Turkey, with prevalence ranging from 19.6 to 420/100,000h. It is also common in Asian countries (Iran, Iraq, Japan, China.) 2.1 and 19.5/100,000h. In Europe, with a decreasing South-North frequency gradient, Portugal, Spain, Italy and France: 1.5 to 15.9/100,000h, Sweden, the United Kingdom and Germany: 0.3 to

4.9/100,000h. In North America: 5.2 cases/100,000h[12]. In North African countries, particularly the Maghreb, MB is relatively common and is the 2nd most common inflammatory disease of the central nervous system after multiple sclerosis.[ème]

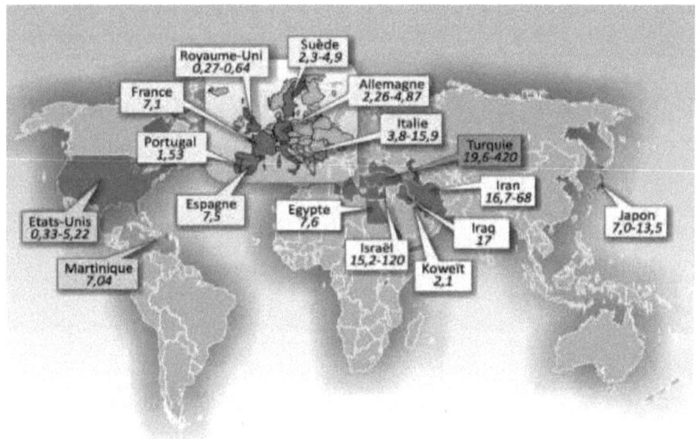

Figure 2: Worldwide prevalence of Behçet's disease. Figures represent prevalence rates per 100,000 population. [12]

2°) Age and gender :

Other epidemiological features of this disease are the relatively early age of onset. In the majority of cases, the average age at diagnosis is around 30, while it is rare before the age of 15 and exceptional after the age of 50. A predominance of males (3 males to 1 female) has been described in the literature[12] . Male MB tends to be more severe.

IV) ETIOPATHOGENESIS

The aetiopathogenesis of MB remains unexplained. Pathophysiological data suggest that the inflammatory reaction in MB results from a disruption of the innate and adaptive immune response in genetically predisposed individuals, and in the presence of environmental factors, such as an infectious agent that secondarily provokes, by cross-reactivity, the proliferation of T cells that are autoreactive towards human HSP. This results in the activation of T lymphocytes in peripheral blood and inflammatory sites (13,14) .

1°) Infectious hypothesis (15,16)

Several infectious agents have been incriminated in the pathogenesis of the inflammatory process of MB in a genetically susceptible individual. These antigens from viruses of the Herpes family, or from bacteria belonging to Streptococcus species, show strong homologies with human proteins such as human HSP, leading to a cross immune response in genetically predisposed individuals. These data have not

In addition, the lack of efficacy of anti-herpes treatment makes this hypothesis implausible. Poor oral hygiene and the presence of recurrent mouth ulcers during the course of MB have suggested an oral bacterial infection, particularly streptococcal. Improvements in MB after antistreptococcal treatment have been reported. In addition to infectious agents, it has also been suggested that the endogenous microbiota is potentially involved in the pathogenesis of MB. In particular, a poorer and dysbiotic salivary and faecal microbial community has been described in MB compared with healthy controls. Reduced microbial diversity was associated with lower production of butyrate, one of the most representative short-chain fatty acids (SCFAs) capable of affecting T regulatory cells (Tregs).

2°) Heat shock proteins [17,18, 20]

HSPs (Heat Shock Proteins) are highly conserved proteins found in a latent state in microorganisms (bacteria, viruses, etc.) and mammalian tissues. HSPs can be induced by infection, trauma, heat, UV-B, hypoxia and cold. These proteins are powerful activators of T lymphocytes. They are named according to their molecular weight in kilodalton (kDa), HSP60 for mammals and HSP65 proteins for microorganisms. High levels of anti-HSP60/65 antibodies were observed in the blood and cerebrospinal fluid of MB patients with neurological involvement. Anti-HSP-65 antibodies cross-reacting with oral mucosal homogenates and oral streptococci have been reported in MB. These data suggest that these and other peptides (bacteria, viruses, etc.) are the antigens that trigger the immune process in MB.Recent data on the physiology of the innate immune system and the description of Toll-like receptors (TLRs) and HSP-60 as a ligand for TLR-2 and TLR-4 suggest that HSP-60 represents an endogenous 'danger' signal for the innate immune system, with rapid release of inflammatory cytokines.

3°) Genetic hypothesis

The preponderance of MB in the Mediterranean basin and along the Silk Road suggests the existence of a genetic susceptibility[12] . Studies have shown that HLA-B51 is the main genetic susceptibility factor[20] . The relative risk of developing MB in carriers of the HLA-B51 allele is 5 to 6 times higher than in the general population[12] .Despite the recent identification of several susceptibility genes. HLA-B∗51 remains the most important genetic factor in Behçet's disease. It has been shown that the prevalence of HLA-B∗51 differs according to groups phenotype in the same patient population. HLA-B∗51 shows an epistatic interaction with the endoplasmic reticulum aminopeptidase (ERAP) 1 allele encoding the Hap10 allotype. The ERAP1 association was absent in individuals lacking HLA-B*51. Individuals carrying HLA-B*51 and also homozygous for the haplotype had an increased risk of disease compared with those without either risk factor (p = 4.80 × 10-20, OR 10.96, 95% CI 5.91 to 20.32). The ERAP1 allotype associated with Behçet's disease has been shown to have low peptide clearance activity. These data suggest that a hypoactive ERAP1 allotype contributes to the risk of Behçet's disease by modifying the peptides available to bind to HLA-B*51. In addition to HLA-B*51, other HLA class 1 alleles, such as A*26, B*15 and B*27, have been identified as genetic susceptibility factors for MB[20] . In addition to HLA and ERAP1, a series of GWAS have also identified MB susceptibility loci at several genes linked to innate and adaptive immune function. Levels of T helper (Th1 and Th17) related cytokines, such as IL-12, interferon (IFN)-γ, IL-17A, IL- 17F, IL-22, IL-23, IL-8, and GM-CSF) have also been extensively studied[21] .

Thus, a genetic predisposition to MB is associated with alterations in the functioning of the adaptive and innate immune system (neutrophils, NK cells, Tγδ), resulting in the release of reactive oxidative species (ROS) by these cells contributing to tissue damage, vasculitis and endothelial cell dysfunction with NO release, inflammation and thrombosis. Histopathological analysis has shown that arteries and veins are infiltrated by neutrophils and lymphocytes, leading to endothelial cell dysfunction and vascular inflammation in MB patients[21] .

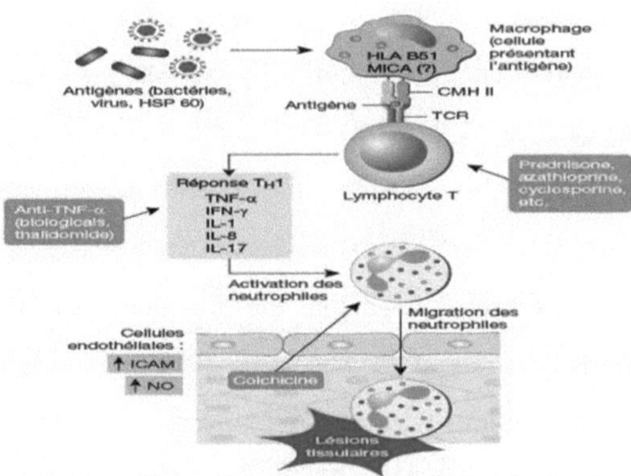

Figure 3: Hypothetical model of the pathogenesis of Behçet's disease (Fig 3).

Under the influence of viral and bacterial antigens, and in the context of a genetic predisposition, there is a Th1 stimulation which leads to activation of neutrophils and endothelial cells, resulting in tissue damage. The different classes of drugs used in Behçet's disease and their therapeutic targets are indicated by the blue frames.·(22, 23)

TCR: T cell receptor; HSP: heat shock protein 60; MHC II: molecule of the major histocompatibility complex class I; TNF-: tumor necrosis factor; IFN-: interferon-; IL: interleukin; ICAM-1: intercellular adhesion molecule-1; NO: nitric oxide. Neurobehçet includes both intracerebral (parenchymal involvement) and extracerebral forms. Extra-cerebral forms, dominated by venous thrombosis, are seen in 10 to 40% of cases of MB. The pathogenic mechanism is not well understood. However, several studies suggest endothelial dysfunction secondary to an inflammatory process in the development of thrombosis[(24)] (Endothelin-1, ICAM-1, VCAM-1, P and E selectins, etc.).

V) ANATOMOPATHOLOGY [25]

The histopathological lesion is a perivascular inflammation affecting vessels of all sizes, arteries, veins and venules. The anatomical substrate common to all these conditions is a predominantly venular vasculitis. These lesions are characterised by perivascular lymphocytic and monocytic infiltration with or without fibrin deposition in the vascular wall associated with tissue necrosis. Significant neutrophil infiltration may also be seen, especially in early lesions.

VI) SYSTEMIC MANIFESTATIONS

A) Mucocutaneous manifestations :

1) Mouth ulcers :

• Oral ulcerations are the most frequent manifestation (99%) and are the first signs of the disease in 80% of cases, but may occur several months or even years after the other systemic manifestations. May be single or multiple most often spontaneous in onset (Fig 4), are characterised by recurrent episodes of rounded mouth ulcers with erythematous margins covered with a yellowish-white or greyish fibrinous exudate (1-3 cm in diameter)[26] . The preferred site for these mouth ulcers is the inside of the lips and cheeks, the gingivolabial fold, the edge or frenulum of the tongue, the floor of the mouth, the palate, the tonsils and the pharynx. Generally little or no pain, often

The diagnosis of Behçet's disease requires the presence of recurrent oral aphthosis with more than 3 episodes per year[27] .

• Oral aphthae may be accompanied by genital aphthae in 60 to 65% of cases and are highly suggestive of MB when they are observed during the inflammatory phase or in the scarred state in the form of depigmented scars, allowing a retrospective diagnosis. In men, they frequently occur on the scrotum, rarely on the penis; in women, on the labia minora and majora, vagina and cervix[28] .

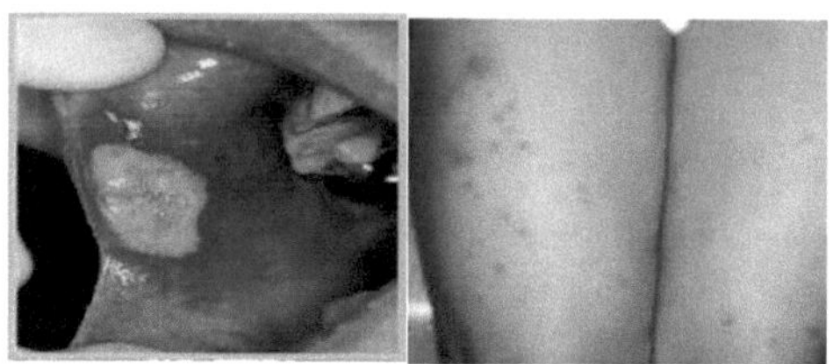

Figure 4 Mouthulcer

Figure 5 Pseudofolliculitis

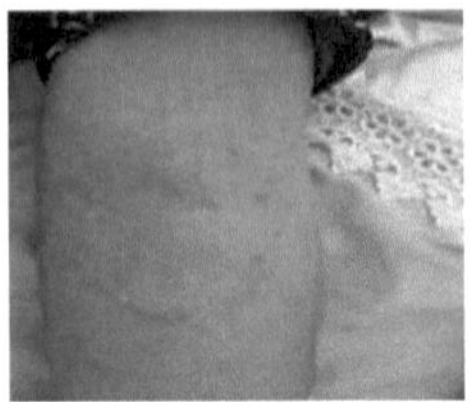

Figure 6 Pathergy test

2) Other skin manifestations include :

- Pseudofolliculitis are papulopustular lesions (Fig 5) not centred on a hair.
- Cutaneous hyperreactivity, also known as the pathergy test (Fig 6), secondary to attacks on the epithelium at the injection site, of perfusion, superficial scratch or intradermal reaction to various antigens. The test is carried out using a 20-22 gauge needle, penetrated obliquely into the skin to a depth of 5 mm, and injected with physiological serum.

erythematous, more than 2 mm in diameter, at the site of the bite, 48 hours later; a small pustule may appear at the top. The sensitivity of this test is reduced by the use of disposable equipment and skin disinfection.Hypodermal nodules are often encountered, in the form of recurrent erythema nodosum, which is frequently described in this disease[28] .

B) Ophthalmological symptoms

Ocular manifestations are serious and have a major impact on visual prognosis. They form part of the diagnostic criteria for Behçet's disease [4,5, 6] . Behçet's disease is an inflammatory lesion which progresses in recurrent attacks, generally starting on one side and which may become bilateral over the course of the disease. It may affect the anterior and posterior chambers of the eye (uveitis) 32 to 53

(Fig 7), as well as the retina (retinal vasculitis). Uveitis may be inaugural in 10-20% of cases, but generally appears 2-3 years after oral aphthosis[29] . The clinical aspects of ocular involvement are variable, fleeting and acute in onset, marked by a drop in visual acuity, peri-keratotic ocular redness, moderate periorbital pain associated with photophobia and lacrimation[29] .

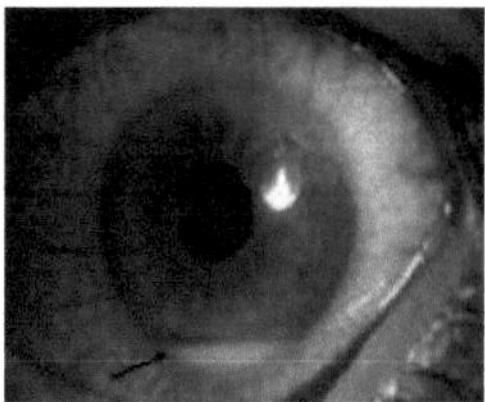

Figure 7: Red eye in acute anterior uveitis with hypopyon (arrow)[29] .

Examination[30] :

Anterior veitis: there is a vitreous tyndall which is very characteristic of inflammatory activity, inflammatory adhesions between the iris and the lens (iridocrystalline synechiae) responsible for deformation.

pupil. When a hypopyon is found in approximately 15% of cases, this is a sign of highly suggestive of the disease and generally correlated with a severe visual prognosis.Posterior uveitis, also known as choroiditis, is the most serious form of uveitis and can be life-threatening. The main lesion is arterial and venous vasculitis. It is present in half of all cases. It may be focal, multifocal or diffuse, and manifests itself in the form of yellowish-white, haemorrhagic foci of retinitis. Retinal vasculitis frequently manifests itself as occlusive periphlebitis in the form of whitish perivascular mantles, sometimes associated with haemorrhages.

C) Joint manifestations :

Articular manifestations are frequent, described in about 50% of cases according to study series[31] . They usually occur early[32] . They may also precede the other manifestations of the disease by several years. Characterised by a polymorphous and recurrent clinical course. The symptoms are arthralgia and/or arthritis in various forms - monoarthritis, oligoarthritis or polyarthritis - affecting mainly the large joints (hips, knees, ankles, wrists and elbows)[27] . Treatment is generally favourable and the disease usually heals without sequelae.

D) Vascular manifestations :

The vascular manifestations of Behçet's disease are dominated by venous involvement (deep and superficial). The location of these venous thromboses varies: lower limbs, vena cava (superior or inferior), cerebral veins, suprahepatic or portal veins. The thrombophilia of venous thrombosis in Behçet's disease is secondary to inflammation rather than to a coagulation disorder [33,34] .

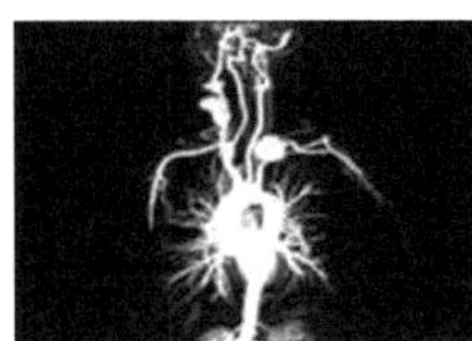

Figure 8: Multiple aneurysms (left subclavian, right common carotid, right internal carotid) in a patient with vasculo-Behçet.

Arterial involvement (arterial aneurysms (Fig 8) and arterial occlusions) is less frequent, occurring in 5 to 10% of cases. It may affect all territories, with a predominance of the abdominal aorta and arteries. pulmonary disease. Arterial involvement is the most serious aspect of the disease. The prognosis in the event of aneurysm rupture is extremely severe, with a high mortality rate of around 30-40% [35,36].

E) Cardiac manifestations

Cardiac involvement is rare. All tunics may be affected. Pericarditis is most often inaugural and recurrent. Coronary involvement may be isolated or associated with pericarditis, and frequently manifests itself as a myocardial infarction[27] .

F) Manifestations of other organs :

1) Digestive: Aphthous lesions can occur in all segments of the digestive tract (oesophagus, stomach, intestine or anal margin) (Fig 9). The risk of these lesions is digestive perforation, especially in ileocecal lesions[27] .

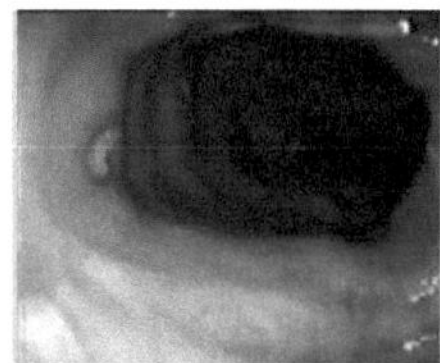

Figure 9: Multiple apthoid lesions in the ileum of a female patient. with entero-Behçet [37]

2) Renal :

Very rare, dominated by amyloid nephropathy[38] . It occurs in patients who have had the disease for many years and are poorly controlled.

3) Pleuropulmonary :

Pleuropulmonary involvement is exceptional. The most common are pulmonary artery aneurysms, pulmonary embolism and infarction,
life-threatening pleural effusion and pulmonary haemorrhage, especially in the case of sudden, large haemoptysis [38,39] .

4) Testicular or epididymal**:** (orchi-epididymitis)[40] .

Testicular involvement is less frequent, and may occur in the course of a Behçet's disease.

G) Neurological manifestations or Neuro-Behçet (NB).

Neurological involvement in Behçet's disease, commonly known as Neuro-Behçet (NB), is relatively common[12] . It varies from 5% to over 50% depending on the series. It occurs most often 4 to 5 years after the diagnosis of BD, concomitantly in 7.5% and inaugurally in 3 to 30% of cases[12] . The clinical and radiological polymorphism involved in diagnosing NB is difficult, especially in inaugural forms. NB criteria have been proposed and constantly re-evaluated by the Behçet Disease Study Group[41] (Table 1).

Table 1: Characteristics of 5 classification systems for Behçet's disease.[3,4]

Variables	Criteria					
	Mason and Barnes	O'Duffy	JBDRC 1974	JBDRC 1987	International Study Group	International Criteria For Behçet's Disease
Year from publication	1969	1974	1974	1987	1990	2013
classification elements						
Oral aphthosis (AB)	Major	Major	Major	Major	Mandatory	2 points
Genitalaphthosis (GA)	Major	Major	Major	Major	Optional	2 points
Eye damage	Major	Major	Major	Major	Optional	2 points
Skin damage	Major	Major	Major	Major	Optional	1 point
Positive patch test					Optional	1 point
Arthritis/arthralgia	Minor	Major	Minor	Minor		
Vascular damage			Minor	Minor		1 point
Thrombophlebitis	Minor					
Cardiovascular disease	Minor					
Neurological damage	Minor	Major	Minor	Minor		1 point
Digestive disorders	Minor		Minor	Minor		
Orchi-epididymitis			Minor	Minor		
Family history	Minor					
Conditions of	3 items	Shape	Shape	Shape	AB and	at least 4
filling of	major ;	complete :	complete :	complete :	minus 2	points
criteria	2 items major	AB or AG and 2 others	4 items major	4 items major	items optional	

and 2 minor items

major items

Incomplete form: AB and one other major item; AG and 1 other item major

Incomplete form: 3 major items; eye damage and one other item major

Incomplete form: 3 items major; 2 major and 2 minor items; eye damage and one other item major; 2 minor items

JBDRC: Japanese Behçet's Disease Research Committee*Optional element.A consensus has been reached on the diagnosis of these neurological forms international in 2014[6]

1- Neuro-Behçet defined :

A. Patients meeting the international diagnostic criteria for MB

B. Objective clinical neurological syndrome associated with Behçet's disease and associated with neuroimaging and/or CSF analysis abnormalities.

C. No aetiological alternative to the disorders presented

2- Probable neuro-Behçet :

A. Objective neurological syndrome as defined in 1, but in a patient without does not meet all the diagnostic criteria for MB

B. Uncharacteristic neurological syndrome in a patient with definite MB.

NB is frequently manifested by parenchymal involvement preferentially the mesodiencephalic junction, occurring in the form of neurovascular (venous or arterial). Involvement of the peripheral nervous system is exceptional and remains the subject of debate.

1) **Parenchymal involvement:** "classic" parenchymal neuro-Behçet. Parenchymal involvement is the most common form of NB, accounting for 29% to 98% of neurological manifestations[5] . Clinically, this entity includes an inflammatory central neurological syndrome not explained by another neurological condition. Men tend to be more affected than women, with a median age of 30 to 40 years, and MB that has been evolving for at least five years[42] . The clinical picture may be acute or progressive, often marked by headaches in half the cases, unilateral or bilateral pyramidal syndrome, cerebellar ataxia and sphincter disorders. Diffuse involvement of the cerebral parenchyma can also take the form of meningoencephalitis, especially if the onset is acute, with neuropsychiatric signs, psychomotor slowing, behavioural changes and even a confusional syndrome, posing a diagnostic problem in "inaugural" neurological forms of MB [43,44] . In such situations, several differential diagnoses are raised. Rigorous questioning and clinical examination in search of signs or scars suggestive of MB that have gone unnoticed will help in the diagnosis of NB. Other symptoms are also observed, but are rare: sensory disorders, focal or generalised epilepsy, damage to the cranial pairs, extrapyramidal syndrome (Parkinsonian syndrome, focal dystonia, chorea) [45,46] . Brain imaging assists in the diagnosis of NB (Fig 10, 11, 12, 13). Parenchymal lesions are mainly studied using magnetic resonance imaging (MRI), which remains the reference technique in this disease[47] . Lesions are generally asymmetric, most often distributed in the diencephalon and brain stem.

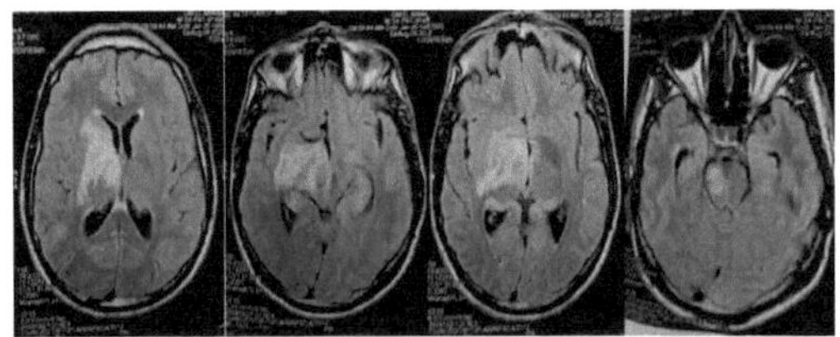

Figure 10:Figure 11Figure 12Figure 13

Brain MRI: axial section, Flair sequence showing unilateral infiltration in the form of a "thalamo-mesencephalic flow" along the corticospinal tract.

a) Pseudotumour forms

Neuro-Behçet patients with a tumour-like form on imaging cerebral damage are rare, reported in the literature as isolated cases. A series has recently been published[(48)] , and the clinical picture is severe, most often characterised by unilateral pyramidal damage with functional impotence. It poses a problem of differential diagnosis, mainly with tumour pathologies (glioblastomas or lymphomas) or infectious pathologies, essentially tubercular abscesses[(49)] . They may be inaugural or occur during the course of the disease. In the absence of a stereotactic biopsy for the purpose of a definitive diagnosis, it is advisable to carry out radiological examinations using CT and/or MRI of the brain (Fig 14, 15, 16). Partial or total reversibility of lesions under treatment with significant clinical improvement appears to be a characteristic feature of Neuro-Beçet[(49)] .

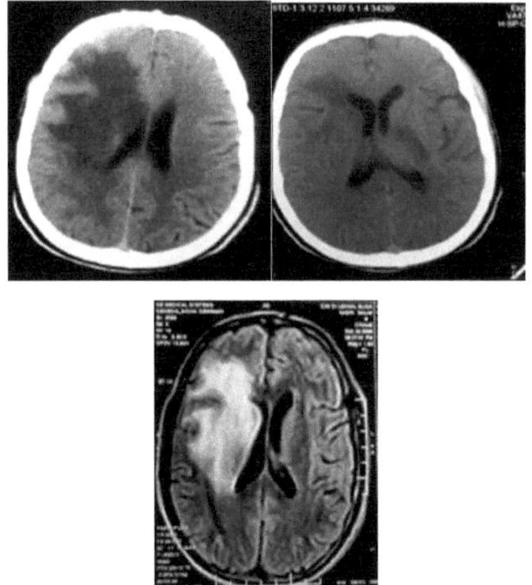

Figure 14 SPC brain CTFigure **15**SPC brain CT Figure16 Brain MRIT2 Before treatment 15 days after treatment

Imaging: SPC CT and brain MRI: NB pseudotumour form.

b) Spinal cord injuries

Spinal cord involvement predominates in the cervical cord. These lesions are often an extension of damage to the lower part of the brain stem[50] (Fig 17). Isolated myelitis is exceptional[50] . The phenotype is transverse myelitis with a sensory level, pyramidal syndrome and sphincter disorders. These clinical and radiological features are not specific to the disease. They pose a problem of differential diagnosis with other inflammatory pathologies, particularly multiple sclerosis.

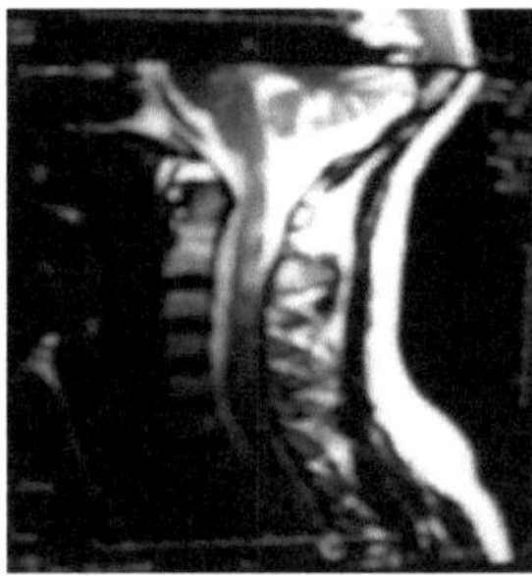

Figure 17: T2 spinal cord MRI, hyper signals in the cervical spinal cord

2) Neurovascular or extra-parenchymal damage

Extra-parenchymal damage may be venous or arterial. Cerebral venous thrombosis is the most common.

c) Venous thrombosis

All venous sinuses may be involved, in particular the superior, inferior, transverse and right sinuses [42,46] (Fig 18,19). The clinical manifestations of cerebral venous thrombosis vary. The onset is usually subacute, within a few days, and is marked by the following signs intracranial hypertension headache, papilledema associated with vomiting and paralysis of the external oculomotor nerve. A motor deficit or a focal or generalised epileptic seizure may also be observed. [51].

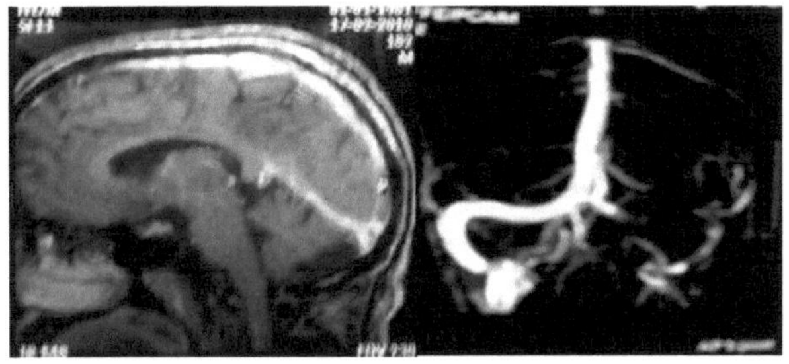

Figure 18: Cerebral MRI: T1 sagittal slice

Figure 19 : MRI angiogram, left lateral sinus thrombosis of the superior longitudinal sinus

d) Arterial disease

Cerebral arterial damage is much rarer (Fig 20) in NB series than venous damage(52) . The mechanism may be occlusion or aneurysm of arteries destined for the brain (53,54) . Aneurysms are at risk of rupture and are the main cause of death(54) .

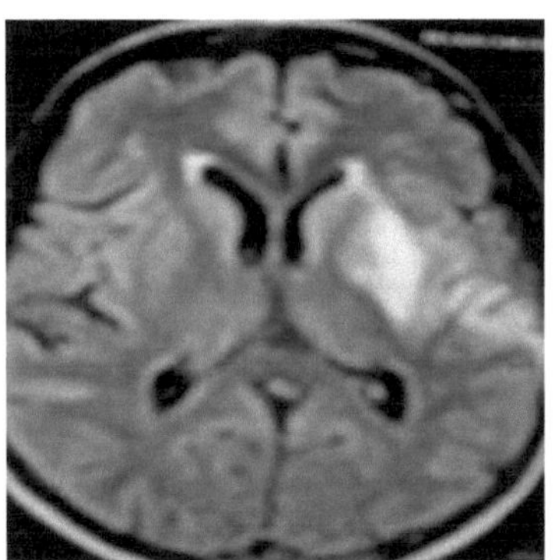

Figure 20: Axial MRI, Flair showing ischemic stroke

3) Additional examinations

a) Neuroimaging

Magnetic resonance imaging is the gold standard for this pathology[47] . At present, NB in its various parenchymal and vascular clinical forms requires investigation by magnetic resonance imaging (MRI), angioimaging sequences, etc., as well as by magnetic resonance imaging (MRI). (angioscanner, angio-MRI). It is superior to CT because of its greater sensitivity and specificity. It is of vital importance in cases of NB where cerebral CT has been shown to be normal. Cerebral MRI allows better detection of lesions located in the diencephalon, basal ganglia, walls of the third ventricle, optic tracts and especially the brainstem[55] .

➢ Exploration protocol

✓ Brain: axial and coronal sections T2, Flair, T2*, Diffusion, T1 -/+ gado sequences.

✓ Spinal cord: Sagittal and axial sections, Sequences: T2, STIR and T1 - / + gado

✓ Cerebral veins:AngioMR and Angioscanner

In classic parenchymal NB, lesions are asymmetric, multiple and of different sizes in several areas of the central nervous system. The most common pathognomonic sites for NB are, in descending order, the mesodiencephalic junction (46%), the ponto-bulbar area (40%), the hypothalamic-thalamic area (23%) and the basal ganglia (18.5%). The medulla oblongata is rarely affected (4.6%). However, magnetic resonance imaging may be normal in around 10-20% of cases, particularly in acute forms, where abnormalities may appear. secondary to MRI [56,57] .

Early initiation of treatmentimmunosuppressive therapy can completely eliminate the lesions at imaging correlates with clinical remissions. At a distance from an attack, and in progressive forms, atrophy of the brainstem is sometimes observed, which may represent an a posteriori marker of NB[56] , without associated cerebral atrophy and with a follow-up of more than one year.

Periventricular white matter lesions, unlike demyelinating pathologies such as multiple sclerosis (MS), are not very suggestive of NB (56).

In cases of extra-parenchymal involvement, the reference imaging technique is MRI angiography, which can reveal venous thrombosis as well as arterial complications[47] . Venous MRI angiography can show thrombosis of the superior longitudinal sinus, the two lateral sinuses and the right sinus, with dilatation of the cortical veins[42] .

b) Data from cerebrospinal fluid analysis.

Analysis of cerebrospinal fluid is essential in all inflammatory diseases of the central nervous system. NB is often associated with aseptic lymphocytic meningitis, which is very characteristic of the diagnosis when there is no extra-neurological involvement. In this case, study of the CSF shows a predominantly lymphocytic pleocytosis of 30 to 50 elements/mm3 for lymphocytic meningitis, with hyperproteinorachy at 0.6 g/l. The existence of ephemeral oligoclonal IgG synthesis in the CSF is not specific and is also found in many other inflammatory diseases of the CNS (MS, neurosarcoidosis, neurolupus, etc.). It is not generally found in extra-parenchymal forms[5] .

4) Positive diagnosis of NB.

➢ **1ére situation :**

When MB is known to exist in a patient treated in dermatology or internal medicine for recurrent aphthosis, or in ophthalmology for uveitis, followed by the secondary appearance of neurological signs, it is easy to link the symptoms to MB.

➢ **2ème situation:** When MB is unknown; the diagnosis is made in the presence of a characteristic neurological picture:

✓ Cerebral thrombophlebitis

✓ Stroke in young people

✓ Recurrent neurological symptoms of the central nervous system in a young male subject.

✓ Imaging, particularly cerebral MR, can help in the diagnosis.

5) Evolution: Neuro-Behçet evolves in several forms

✓ Thrust-remission.

✓ Secondary progressive forms (after a relapsing-remitting phase),

✓ Primary progressive forms.

In the Turkish cohort of Siva et al(51) , the course of the disease was as follows: 73.7% of patients had relapses and 26.3% were progressive.

In the absence of treatment, recurrences are frequent (around 30%), particularly in diencephalic and brainstem disorders (58,59) .

6) Prognostic factors: The poor prognostic factors (42,58) , involving the vital prognosis and/or leaving incapacitating after-effects are:

✓ Aseptic meningitis, particularly in patients with a higher cellularity;

✓ Parenchymal involvement, particularly in the extensive form diencephalo-mesencephalic.

✓ Arterial damage, particularly ischaemic stroke.

✓ At least two relapses per year.

✓ Impaired general condition when NB is diagnosed.

✓ Relapses under treatment;

✓ A progressive form (primary or secondary).

✓ general complications (decubitus complications, pulmonary and skin superinfections).

7) Differential diagnosis of Neuro-Behçet

In inflammatory diseases of the central nervous system, a number of differential diagnoses have been suggested (60,61) :

✓ Infectious pathologies: viral meningoencephalitis (herpes), bacterial meningoencephalitis (tuberculosis and atypical mycobacteria, rhombencephalitis with Listeria monocytogenes). The benefits of
LCS study.

✓ Inflammatory diseases Multiple sclerosis; Neurosarcoidosis; Neurolupus ;

✓ Ischaemic strokes.

✓ Brain tumours (pseudotumour forms).

a) NeuroBehçet or Multiple Sclerosis

➢ **Arguments in favour of NB :**

✓ Sex: Male > Female

✓ The most typical symptoms are

- Headaches (> 50% of cases),
- Uni- or bilateral pyramidal syndrome (50-90%),
- Cerebellar ataxia, sphincter disorders (25-40%).
- Sensory disorders (< 40%),
- Epilepsy (5-10%),
- Phasic disorders (5-10%).
- NORB, isolated or associated with other symptoms are rare in NB (0.6 to 2%).

✓ Involvement of the cranial pairs is also rare.

✓ An extrapyramidal syndrome is very rare (parkinsonian syndrome, focal dystonia, chorea) and may sometimes be indicative of parenchymal damage.

➢ **Inaugural signs of multiple sclerosis (MS)**[62]

Étude	Optic neuritis	Motor deficit	Sensitive disorders	Brain stem	Ataxia	Sphincter disorders
McAlpine	22%	40 %	21 %	17 %	-	5 %
Weinshenker	17,2%	20,1%	45,4%	12,9%	13,2%	-
Comi	31,7%	34,1%	48,3%	2,6%	-	-

Table 2. Inaugural signs of multiple sclerosis [62]

➢ **Uveitis**

✓ In Behçet's disease, uveitis is the second most frequent manifestation, generally developing within 2 to 3 years of the aphthae and inaugurating in 10 to 20% of patients[29] . It is usually bilateral, progressing in successive flare-ups or on a more chronic basis. It affects the anterior and posterior compartments separately or simultaneously[29] .

✓ In MS, uveitis is very rare (0.8% to 14% of cases)[63] .

➢ **Imaging, in particular cerebral MRI, reveals the following in NB :**

Lesions in NB are predominantly located in the brainstem and tend to be anterior. The most frequently found abnormality is unilateral infiltration of the internal capsule, thalamus and mesencephalon, in the form of a "thalamo-mesencephalic flow", along the corticospinal tract. Another feature of these lesions is their reversibility, according to studies[49] :

✓ 40% of lesions disappear completely on follow-up MRI scans,

✓ 35% decrease in size

✓ 25% remain unchanged;

Brainstem atrophy is one of the manifestations of chronic NB. Brainstem atrophy without cortical atrophy is a specific sign of NB (specificity of 96.5%

and low sensitivity) [47,64] . In contrast, MS lesions involve the floor of the fourth ventricle in the brainstem and the middle cerebellar peduncle. Involvement of the periventricular white matter and corpus callosum, the oval appearance and the perpendicular arrangement of the lesions to the lateral ventricles are arguments in favour of MS. Subtentorial lesions, particularly of the cerebellum and medulla oblongata, are more suggestive of MS than of NB. [65]. The CSF is abnormal in 70 to 80% of cases of parenchymal involvement of the NB. according to studies [42,58, 66] .

✓ Protein levels are often moderately high, sometimes reaching 1 g/l.

✓ The presence of oligoclonal IgG bands is very rare, and when they do occur, they disappear rapidly, unlike in MS.

✓ CSF is typically hypercellular with hypercytosis, generally consisting of an initial exclusive polynucleosis replaced by lymphocytosis at a later stage.

In MS, the number of cells in the CSF rarely exceeds 35 (mainly lymphocytes).

Table 3: Comparative inaugural clinical signs between multiple sclerosis and Neuro-Behçet.

	SEP	NB
gender	Women+++	Men+++
clinic		
Frequent initial signs and symptoms	Optic neuritis Internuclear ophthalmoplegia Sensory disorders Spinal cord injury Pyramidal syndrome Syndrome cerebellar	Headache Syndrome pyramidal Syndrome cerebellar Cranial nerve damage
Signs and Rare symptoms	Headache Cranial nerve damage	Optic neuritis Sensory disorders Spinal cord injury Internuclear ophthalmoplegia

Table 4: Comparative MRI scans between MS and NB

	SEP	Neuro-Behçet
Brain MRI lesions.		
Periventricular Subcortical Brain stem Cerebellum Spinal cord	+++ ++ ++ Small, ++ ++	+ - Large and diffuse + Rare
CSF		
Profile inflammatory Bands oligoclonal	+ +++ 90% Even 100/%.	+ Present but short-lived.

b) Neuro-Behçet or Sarcoidosis

The neurological manifestations of sarcoidosis are a common differential diagnosis of NB, and are difficult to distinguish. Ophthalmological manifestations (uveitis and retinal vasculitis) may also occur in sarcoidosis. In such cases, it is essential to look for the more specific systemic signs of this disease, in particular mediastinal adenopathy and interstitial lung disease, and to carry out an exhaustive laboratory work-up. However, certain imaging features are unique to neurosarcoidosis, in particular contrast-enhancing leptomeningeal infiltration, as well as dural or intramedullary involvement. Myelitis is common in sarcoidosis and MS and is exceptional in MB(67) .

c) Peripheral nervous system damage in neurobehçet (68,69, 70) .

The occurrence of peripheral neuropathy in MB is rare, if not exceptional. Published cases vary. These include multiple mononeuropathies, axonal sensory or sensitivomotor peripheral polyneuropathies and polyradiculoneuritis. A broad aetiological work-up is required before MB can be considered.

H) Paediatric forms of NeuroBehçet [32,71, 72,] .

Unlike adult neurological diseases, childhood neurological diseases are complex to diagnose and to treat. This makes them one of the most serious problems in paediatric pathology. The average age of onset of the disease is around 8 years, the sex/ratio is the same, with as many boys as girls.unlike in adults, where there is a predominance of males. Clinically it There is no difference between adults and children. Another very In paediatrics, the existence of other affected family members with early onset of the disease is important, suggesting a genetic factor (41, 69, 70).

I) Family forms of MB [24,41, 73]

Familial forms have been described and appear to have an earlier age of onset and to be more severe than sporadic forms. The genetic factor (HLA B51 antigen) appears to be a determining factor. They account for around 5% of MB cases. The risk of any other member of the patient's family being affected in turn is fairly low.

J) MB and Pregnancy [74,75, 76] .

Studies on the influence of pregnancy on MB are controversial. Some studies favour a 70% rate of remission of the disease during pregnancy, others a 15% rate of exacerbation of the disease. However, the majority of studies favour an improvement in the clinical signs of MB during pregnancy. During pregnancy, there is a reduction in immune functions, both cellular and humoral. This could be partly explained by a very high of progesterone, HCG, alpha-fetoprotein and oestrogen, which appears to have an inhibitory effect on immune responses, and a reduction in neutrophil chemotaxis and neutrophil activity. adhesive properties during pregnancy. This process is at the origin of remission of the disease. The rate of pregnancy-related complications (gestational hypertension, gestational diabetes, prematurity, infection, premature rupture of membranes, miscarriage, thromboembolic events) is higher than in the general population.

VII) THERAPEUTIC MANAGEMENT

The complex pathogenesis, polymorphous clinical manifestations, diagnostic difficulty, diversity of clinical forms and recurrent course of MB are the subject of several clinical studies and therapeutic trials with the aim of establishing appropriate therapeutic protocols. All these factors make the therapeutic management of this disease difficult. The aim of treatment is to combat the inflammatory process in order to reduce or eliminate relapses, control mucocutaneous and joint lesions, improve quality of life and prevent the occurrence of irreversible damage, including ocular and neurological damage. Today, the treatment of MB is guided by the severity of the disease and the type of organ affected(77) . In general, colchicine, non-steroidal anti-inflammatory drugs (NSAIDs) and corticosteroids are often sufficient to control the mucocutaneous and joint manifestations of MB. Involvement of other organs, particularly neurological, ocular and gastrointestinal, which may be life-threatening or functionally impaired, requires a more aggressive strategy from the outset, with immunosuppressive drugs.

1) Conventional therapies(78)

• Colchicine :

✓ it is an immunomodulator which acts by inhibiting neutrophil chemotaxis.

✓ Dosage: 1 to 2 mg with a satisfactory response in 60 to 70% of cases of mucocutaneous and joint disorders.

✓ This compound, combined with antiaggregant treatment, has a role in preventing relapses.

• Thalidomide :

✓ It is an immunosuppressant whose mechanism of action remains unknown. in the MB.

✓ Dose: 100mg/d.

✓ Effective on mucocutaneous lesions refractory to colchicine.

✓ Risk of foetopathy

✓ This compound is contraindicated in pregnancy.

- **Corticosteroids :**

Corticosteroids are indicated for neurological and ocular disorders. They may be initiated during acute attacks by daily boluses over 3 to 5 days of methyl prednisolone: bolus: IV 1g/d for 3 to 5 days, then followed up with prednisone: 1mg/kg/d for 6 weeks, then a 10% reduction every 15 days. A maintenance dose of corticosteroid therapy of 10 to 20mg to prevent relapses.

- **Immunosuppressants (IS) :**

SIs facilitate corticosteroid withdrawal but cannot be used on their own. It is advisable to introduce SI at the start of corticosteroid withdrawal. They carry a risk of long-term oncogenicity and are contraindicated in pregnancy and breast-feeding.

The most commonly used SIs :

✓ Cyclophosphamide: 600 mg/m² bolus every 4 weeks, or 50 to 100mg/d orally.

✓ Cyclosporine: 3-5mg/kg/d, rapid onset of action but limited use due to neurotoxicity.

✓ Azathioprine: 2.5 mg/kg/d (2-3 mg/kg/d), or 50 mg/d orally for 2 years.

✓ Methotrexate: 7.5 to 15 mg per week

✓ Chlorambucil: 0.1- 0.2mg/kg/d per os, not used because of the haematological toxicity and oncogenic risk.

- **Anticoagulants :**

The use of anticoagulants is controversial, given that the primary cause of thrombosis is inflammation, but they are still indicated in cases of deep vein and artery thrombosis.

- **Plasmapheresis or iv immunoglobulin :**

This therapy is reserved for severe neurological and ocular disorders.

- **Mycophenolate:** for ocular forms.

2) New therapies (78)

- **Immunomodulating treatments**

✓ Interferon alpha 2a or 2b for treatment-resistant ocular forms.

✓ Inhibition of pro-inflammatory cytokines, anti-TNF alpha (Tumor Necrosis Factor), are indicated in NB when Cyclophosphamide and Azathioprine have failed, infliximab+++ and to a lesser extent.

✓ adalimumab (acts by reducing pro-inflammatory cytokines (the level of of IL6 in the CSF)

- **Anti-IL-1**

Serum IL-1 levels are elevated in MB. Anakinra is an IL-1 receptor antagonist that has been shown to be effective in MB refractory to conventional treatments. More recently, an open-label study showed that gevo-
kizumab, a recombinant human anti-interleukin-1 antibody, was well tolerated and rapidly reduced intraocular inflammation over a long period.

- **Therapies targeting lymphocytes**

✓ Anti-CD20: Rituximab is an anti-CD20 ac which displaces LBs.

✓ Anti-CD52: Alemtuzumab is an anti-CD52 antibody which acts by is LT depletion.

✓ Anti-CD25: Daclizumab is a humanised monoclonal antibody directed against CD25.

✓ Anti-IL-6: IL-6 levels are correlated with MB activity. Tocilizumab, a humanised anti-IL-6 receptor antibody, has marketing authorisation only for moderate to severe forms of refractory active rheumatoid arthritis.

✓ Autograft of haematopoietic stem cells: There have been a few cases of MB treated with myeloablative chemotherapy followed by an autograft of T lymphocyte-depleted haematopoietic stem cells.

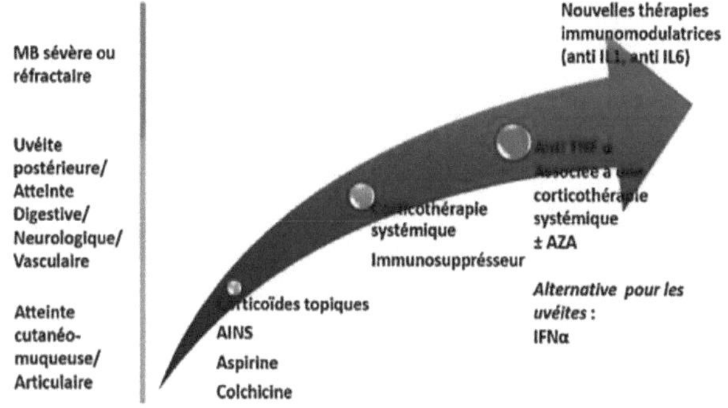

Fig 21: Graduated treatment strategy for Behçet's disease[77] .

AZA: azathioprine; IFN: interferon-alpha; anti-IL-1: interleukin-1 inhibitor; anti-IL-6: interleukin-6 inhibitor; NSAIDs: non-steroidal anti-inflammatory drugs; TNF: Tumor necrosis factor alpha.

3) Proposed treatment for NB

There are currently no recommendations for the treatment of NB, but a consensus of experts[79] has been proposed, which recommends that for the parenchymal form, high-dose corticosteroids should be introduced, starting with a 3-day bolus of methylprednisolone, followed by prednisone 1 mg/kg/d for 4 to 6 weeks. When corticosteroids are withdrawn, an immunosuppressant (Cyclophosphamide IV monthly treatment or oral Azathioprine) should be combined. For cerebral thrombophlebitis, effective anticoagulation was recommended. In the presence of intracranial hypertension (papilledema, CSF hyperpressure), subtractive LP and treatment with acetazolamide are necessary. The favourable response to corticosteroids suggests an inflammatory process in this disease. In order to prevent relapses, they must be introduced early and maintained for a prolonged or even indefinite period of time.

VIII) CONCLUSION

Behçet's disease is a relatively common condition. The etiopathogenesis of the disease remains poorly understood. Genetic and environmental factors play an important role in triggering the inflammatory process of the disease. Both men and women are affected. The clinical phenotype is more severe in men. This condition should be considered when the process is severe and/or recurrent and the patient is from a highly endemic area. There is no biological marker that can be used to establish a definitive diagnosis. Diagnosis is based on clinical criteria that are constantly being revised. The neurological manifestations of MB are dominated by the following disorders of variable clinical presentation. Magnetic resonance imaging (MRI) is the gold standard for this condition. Treatment is not yet well codified, and the prognosis is severe, particularly in cases of neurological or ocular involvement.

REFERENCES

1) Zouboulis CC, Keitel W. A historical review of early descriptions of Adamantiades -Behcet's disease. J Invest Dermatol 2002, 119: 201- 205.

2) Sakane T, Takeno M, Suzuki N, et al. Behçet's disease. New Engl J Med 1999; 341:1284-1291

3) N. Noela et AL, Neurological manifestations of Behçet's disease. Journal of Internal Medicine 35 (2014) 112-120

4) International Study Group for Behçet's disease. Criteria for diagnosis of Behçet's disease. Lacet 1990; 335:1078-80.

5) N. Noel et al / The Journal of Internal Medicine 35 (2014) 112-120

6) Siva A, Altintas A, Saip S. Behc¸ et's syndrome and the nervous system. Curr OpinNeurol 2004; 17:347-57.

7) C. Comarmond , B. Wechsler , P. Cacoub , D. Saadoun∗, treatment of Behcet's disease Revue de médecine interne 35 (2014) 126-138

8) Behçet H. Ueber rezidivierende, aphtöse, durch ein Virus verursachte Geschwüre am Mund, am Auge und an den Genitalien. Dermatol Wochenschr 1937; 105:1152-1157.

9) Mirko D. Grmek, Les maladies à l'aube de la civilisation occidentale, Paris, Payot, 1983, p. 217.

10) Hippocrates (ed. Littré), Œuvres complètes, vol. 3, Paris, Baillière, 1841 (read online [archive]), p. 84

11) Adamantiades B. On a case of iritis with recurrent hypopyon. Ann Oculist (Paris) 1931; 168:271-278.

12) A. Mahr∗, C. Maldini, "epidemiology of Behçet's disease, Revue de médecine interne 35 (2014) 81-89

13) Remmers EF, Cosan F, Kirino Y, Ombrello MJ, Abaci N, Satorius C, et al. Genome-wide association study identifies variants in the MHC class I, IL10 and IL-23R-IL12RB2.regions associated with Behc¸ et's disease. Nat Genet 2010;

42:698-702.

14) Mizuki N, Meguro A, Ota M, Ohno S, Shiota T, Kawagoe T, et al. Genome-wide association studies identify IL23R-IL12RB2 and IL10 as Behc, et's diseasesusceptibility loci. Nat Genet 2010 ; 42:703-6.

15) Mumcu G, Inanc N, Yavuz S, Direskeneli H. The role of infectious agents inthe pathogenesis, clinical manifestations and treatment strategies in Behc, et'sdisease. Clin Exp Rheumatol 2007; 25:27-33.

16) Xiong M, Elson G, Legarda D, Leibovich SJ. Production of vascular endothelial growth factor by murine macrophages: regulation by hypoxia, lactate, and the inducible nitric oxide synthase pathway. American Journal of Pathology. 1998 ; 153(2) :587- 598. [PMC free article] [PubMed] [Google Scholar]

17) Lehner T. The role of heat shock protein, microbial and autoimmune agents inthe aetiology of Behc, et's disease. Int Rev Immunol 1997; 14:21-32.

18) Tanaka T, Yamakawa N, Yamaguchi H, Okada AA, Konoeda Y, Ogawa T, et al.Common antigenicity between Yersinia enterocolitica-derived heat shock pro-tein and the retina, and its role in uveitis. Ophthalmic Res 1996; 28:284-8.

19) Pervin K, Childerstone A, Shinnick T, Mizushima Y, van der Zee R, Hasan A,et al. T cell epitope expression of mycobacterial and homologous human 65-kilodalton heat shock protein peptides in short-term cell lines from patientswith Behcet's disease. J Immunol 1993 ; 151:2273-82.

20) Pablo Guasp ‡ 1, et al; Journal of bioligical chemistry Volume 292, Issue 23, July 2017, Pages 9680-9689, The Behçet's disease-associated variant of the aminopeptidase ERAP1 shapes a low-affinity HLA-B*51 peptidome by differential subpeptidome processingProcessing of the HLA-B*51:08 peptidome by ERAP1

21) Bainan Tong, et al, Front Immunol. Immunopathogenesis of Behcet's Disease Autoimmune and Autoinflammatory Disorders; Volume 10 - 2019.

22) Service d'immunologie et allergie - CHUV (consulted on 05/04/16). Behçet's

disease, [online]. Available at: http://www.immunologyresearch.ch/ial-prof-sante- infomaladies-immunolmaladie-de-behcet.htm.

23) Jean-Philippe Zuber. Pierre-Alexandre. Bart Annette. Leimgruber. François Spertini. Behçet's disease: from Hippocrates to TNF-α antagonists. Articles thématiques : Allergo-immunologie. April 2008.

24) M.H. Houmana. Bel Fekia. Pathophysiology of Behcet's disease. Journal of internal medicine 35 (2014) 90-96.

25) Marshall SE. Behçet's disease. Best Pract Research Clin Rheumatol 2004; 18:291-311.

26) Heriz, A., Hamdi, M. S., Boukhris, I., Azzabi, S., Ben Hassine, L., & Khalfallah, N. Mucocutaneous manifestations during Behçet's disease: a retrospective study of 79 cases. La Revue de Médecine Interne, 36, A92. doi:10.1016/j.revmed.2015.03.054.

27) Zeidan, M. J., Saadoun, D., Garrido, M., Klatzmann, D., Six, A., & Cacoub, P. (2016). Behçet's disease physiopathology: a contemporary review. Autoimmunity Highlights,
7(1). doi : 10.1007/s13317-016-0074-1.

28) Sakane, T., Takeno, M., Suzuki, N., & Inaba, G. (1999). Behçet's Disease. New England Journal of Medicine, 341(17), 1284-1291. doi : 10.1056/nejm199910213411707

29) H. Zeghidia, D. Saadounb, B. Bodaghia. Ocular manifestations of Behçet's disease. Revue de médecine interne 35 (2014) 90-96.

30) Tugal-Tutkun I. Behcet's disease. In: Gupta A, Gupta V, Herbort CP, Khairallah M, editors. Uveitis,text and imaging. Eds Jaypee; 2009. p. 397-413

31) Davatchi F, Chams-Davatchi C, Shams H, et al. Adult Behcet's disease in Iran : analysis of 6075 patients. Int J Rheum Dis . 2016 ; 19(1) :95-103.

32) Piram M, Koné-Paut I. Behçet's disease in children. Rev Médecine Interne. Feb 2014 ; 35(2):121-5.

33) Al Dalaan A.N., et al.1994. Behcet's disease in Saudi Arabia. J Rheumatol

21 : 658- 661.
34) Wechsler B., Piette J.C., Conard J., Lê Thi Huong D., Blétry O., Godeau P. 1987. Deep vein thrombosis in Behçet's disease. Presse Med 16: 661- 664.
35) Bartlett S.T., McCarthy W.J., Palmer A.S., Flinn W.R., Bergan J.J., Yao J.S.T. 1988. Multiple aneurysms in Behçet's disease. Arch Surg : 1004-1008.
36) Christensen P.A., Tvedegaard E., Strandgaard S., Thomsen B.S.1997. Behçet's syndrome presenting with peripheral arterial aneurysms. Scand J Rheumatol 26 : 386-388.
37) zaghloul Rachid. Les anévrismes de l'aorte abdominale au cours d la maladie de Behçet.Mémoire de fin de spécialité. Faculty of medicine of pharmacy of Fez.June 2015, page 26
38) Hamza M, Ben Maiz H, Ben Ayed H. Behçet's disease with renal manifestation. A About a case followed for 6 years. Sem Hôp Paris; 1980; 56: 1081-1083.
39) D Montani. Behçet's disease. Rev Mal Respir Actual 2009; 1:160-163.
40) Saadoun, D., & Wechsler, B. (2012). Behçet's disease. EMC - Traité de Médecine AKOS, 7(1), 1-6. doi : 10.1016/s1634-6939(12)49774-5
41) Isabelle KONE-PAUT et AL: Protocole National de Diagnostic et de Soins sur la Maladie de Behçet. December 2019. P : 9.
42) Akman-Demir G, Serdaroglu P, Tasc¸i B. Clinical patterns of neurological involvement
in Behcet's disease: evaluation of 200 patients. Brain 1999; 122:2171-82.
43) Adnan Al-Araji, Desmond P Kidd. Neuro-Behcet's disease: Epidemiology, clinical characteristics, and management. Lancet Neurol 2009; 8:192-204.
44) Wechsler B, Sbaï A, Du-Boutin LT, Duhaut P, Dormont D, Piette JC. Neurological manifestations of Behçet's disease. Rev Neurol (Paris) 2002; 158:926-33.
45) Yücesan C, Isikay CT, Ozay E, Aydin N, Mutluer N.The clinical involvement patterns of neuro-Behçet's disease. Eur J Neurol 2001 ; 8:92.

46) Saadoun D, Wechsler B, Resche-Rigon M, Trad S, Le Thi Huong D, SbaiA, et al. Cerebral venous thrombosis in Behcet's disease. Arthritis Rheum 2009; 61:518-26.

47) Akman-Demir G, Bahar S, Coban O, Tasci B, Serdaroglu P. Cranial MRI in Behc¸ et'sdisease: 134 examinations of 98 patients. Neuroradiology 2003; 45:851-9.

48) Noel N, Hutié M, Wechsler B, Vignes S, Le Thi Huong-Boutin D, Amoura Z, et al.Pseudotumoural presentation of neuro-Behcet's disease: case series and reviewof literature. Rheumatology 2012; 51:1216-25.

49) Ahmad Alfedaghi S, Masters Y, Mourou M, Eshak O. A cerebral mass in a patient with Behçet's disease: about a case report. J Med Case Rep. 2015 Sep 30; 9: 209. [Free PMC Article] [PubMed]

50) Lo Monaco A, La Corte R, Caniatti L, Borrelli M, Trotta F. Neurologicalinvolvement in North Italian patients with Behc¸ et disease. Rheumatol Int 2006; 26 :1113-9.[14]

51) Siva A, Kantarci OH, Saip S, Altintas A, Hamuryudan V, Islak C, et al. Behc¸ et'sdisease: diagnostic and prognostic aspects of neurological involvement. J Neu-rol 2001;248:95-103.

52) S. Rosenstingl1, E. Dupuy1, O. Alves2, B. George2, G. Tobelem1 Behçet's disease revealed by an intracranial aneurysm. Rev Méd Interne 2001; 22: 177-82

53) Y. Krespi, g. Akman-demir, M. Poyraz, B. Tugcu, O. Coban, R. Tuncay, P.Serdaroglu and S. Bahar Cerebral vasculitis and ischaemic stroke in Behcet's disease: report of one case and review of the literature European. Journal of Neurology 2001, 8 : 719±722.

54) Younes Bensaid, Brahim Lekehal, Abbès El Mesnaoui, Zakariyae Bouziane, Nabil S. Arterial complications of Behçet's disease: 47 cases. e-mémoires de l'Académie Nationale de Chirurgie, 2008, 7 (2) : 54-59

55) Ben Haouda.m,Bergaoui. N,Bouhaouala. H,Touzi. M,Ladeb. M.f, Gannzouni. A, Hamza.R Imagerie du Neuro-Behçet. Feuillets de radiologie,

1993 ; vol 33, n°3 :205- 210.
56) Khaled Bouden. A Cherif. O, Boussama. F, Rokbani.l,Daghfous.M.H Contribution of l'imagerie au diagnostic du Neuro-Behçet a propos de 5 cas. La Tunisie médicale, 1999 ; volume 77, N°11 :562-571.
57) Vidaillet.M, Dormont.D Manifestations neurologiques de la maladie de Behçet. Arteres et veines, May and June 1994; vol XIII, n°3 165-170.
58) Kidd D, Steuer A, Denman AM, Rudge P. Neurological complications in Behçet's syndrome. Brain 1999; 122:2183-94.
59) Houman MH, Hamzaoui-B'Chir S, Ben Ghorbel I, Lamloum M, Ben Ahmed M,Abdelhak S, et al [Neurologic manifestations of Behcet's disease: analysis of aseries of 27 patients]. Rev Med Interne 2002; 23:592-606.
60) Siva A, Saip S. The spectrum of nervous system involvement in Behcet's syndrome and its differential diagnosis. J Neurol 2009 ; 256:513-29.
61) Guichard I, Debard A, Cathébras P. Behçet's disease: a common, multifaceted vasculitis. Médecine Thérapeutique. Jav 2010; 16(1) :25-33.
62) Ouallet, B. Brochet Aspects cliniques, physiopathologiques, et thérapeutiques de la sclérose en plaques. EMC-Neurologie 1 (2004) 415-457.
63) Inès Benabdelaziz, Khadija Moalla,Emna Farhat,Zaineb Brahem,Samia Ben Sassi,Faycel Hentati,Mourad Zouari. Uveitis and multiple sclerosis. Revue Neurologique. Volume 171, Supplement 1, April 2015, page A61.
64) El Fekih Mariem, Bedoui Ines, Bissene Douma, Zaouali Jamel, Hajer Derbali, Ridha Mrissa, M. Mansour. Neurology Department, Hôpital militaire principal d'instruction de Tunis, Tunis, Tunisia. NeuroBehçet : interest of brain imaging - 11/04/21 : 0.1016/j.neurol.2021.02.353.
65) Le Page E, Veillard D, Laplaud DA, et al: Oral versus intravenous high-dose methylprednisolone for treatment of relapses in patients with multiple sclerosis (COPOUSEP): A randomised, controlled, double-blind, non-inferiority trial. Lancet 386 (9997) :974-981, 2015. doi : 10.1016/S0140-6736(15)61137-0.
66) Joseph FG, Scolding NJ. Neuro-Behçet's disease in Caucasians: a study of

22 patients. Eur J Neurol 2007; 14:174-80.
67) I. Ben Ghorbel,W. Bensalem,T. Ben Salem,N. Bel Feki,M. Khanfir,F. Saïd,A. Hamzaoui,M. Lamloum,MH Houman. Clinical and radiological manifestations of neurosarcoidosis. A monocentric series of 17 observations. La Revue de Médecine Interne Volume 36, Supplement 1, June 2015, Pages A158-A159.
68) Sana Ben Amor,Faten Bouattay,Asma Nasr,Laïla Ben Algia,Inès Chatti,Mohamed Salah Harzallah,Sofiène Benammou. Polyneuropathy during Behçet's disease. Revue Neurologique. Volume 171, Supplement 1, April 2015, page A148.
69) I.Ben Ghorbel, Z.Ibnelhadj, M.Zouari, et al. Peripheral neuropathy in Behçet's disease. Rev Neurol 2005 ; 161 :218-220.
70) S. Biaz, M. Zahlane, L. Essaadouni Published26 May 2010 Peripheral neuropathy in Behçet's disease: a case report. 10.1016/J. Rev Med .2010.03.259.
71) Laghmari M1, Karim A, Allali F, Elmadani A, Ibrahimy W, Hajjaj Hassouni N, Chkili T, Elmalki Tazi A, Mohcine Z. La maladie de Behçet chez l'enfant, aspects cliniques et évolutifs Agrave ; propos de 13 cas. Journal français d'ophtalmologie. 2002 November, Vol 25, Num 9, pp 904-8.
72) Fettouma Mazari1, Karim Ait Idir2, Leila Boumati1. Diagnostic difficulties of Behçet's disease in children. Paediatric presentation and brief review of the literature. Med Sci 2018; 5(1) :101-103
73) Zouboulis.C Epidemiology of Adamantiades Behçet's disease. Ann.Med.interne, 1999 vol 150, n°6 :488-498
74) S. Ali-Guechi, D. Roula, S. Boughandjioua, N. Boukhris: Behçet's disease and pregnancy: 28 pregnancies in 20 women. Revue de Médecine Interne. Volume 39, Supplement 2, December 2018, page A230.El Hajoui S,
75) Nabil S, Khachani M, Saadi N, Bezad R, Chraïbi C, Alaoui MT : Grossesse chez des patientes ayant une maladie de Behçet. Revue : La Presse médicale : 2002 Janvier 12, Vol 31, Num 1 Pt 1, pp 19-20.

76) Omar Laghzaoui: Impact of immune diseases on pregnancy experience from the Obstetric Gynaecology Department of the Moulay Ismail Military Hospital, Fez, Morocco. Pan Afr Med J. 2016; 24: 38.

77) Comarmond, B. Wechsler, P. Cacoub, D. Saadoun: Treatment of Behçet's disease. Revue de médecine interne 35 (2014) 126-138.

78) B. Wechsler, P. Cacoub, D. Saadouna. Behçet's disease: news in 2014. Revue de médecine interne 35 (2014) 79-80.

79) Consensus proposal: Diagnostic and therapeutic criteria for Neuro Behçet (2010). Pr C.Mhiri (Sfax Tunisia), Pr M.Arezki (Blida Algeria), Pr A. Benomar (CHU Rabat),Pr F.Belahsen CHU Fès),Pr H. ait Benhaddou (CHU Rabat),Pr M. Bouraza (hôpital militaire Rabat) Dr F.Imounan (CHU Rabat) Dr N.Chtaou(CHU Fès) , Dr S.Lytim (CHU Rabat) , Pr M. Yahyaoui (CHU Rabat)

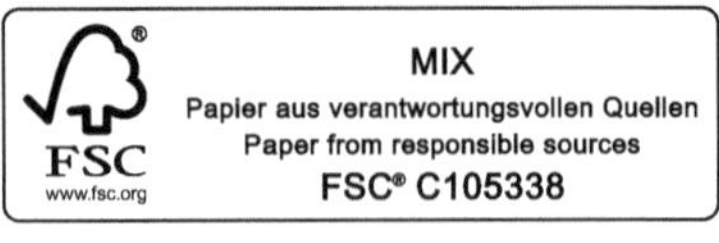

Printed by Books on Demand GmbH, Norderstedt / Germany